PREDIABETES VEGETARIAN RECIPES FOR WEIGHT LOSS

Achieve Healthy Weight Loss and Balance Your Blood Sugar with Our Delicious and Nutritious Collection of Plant-Based Recipes

By Mia Bennett

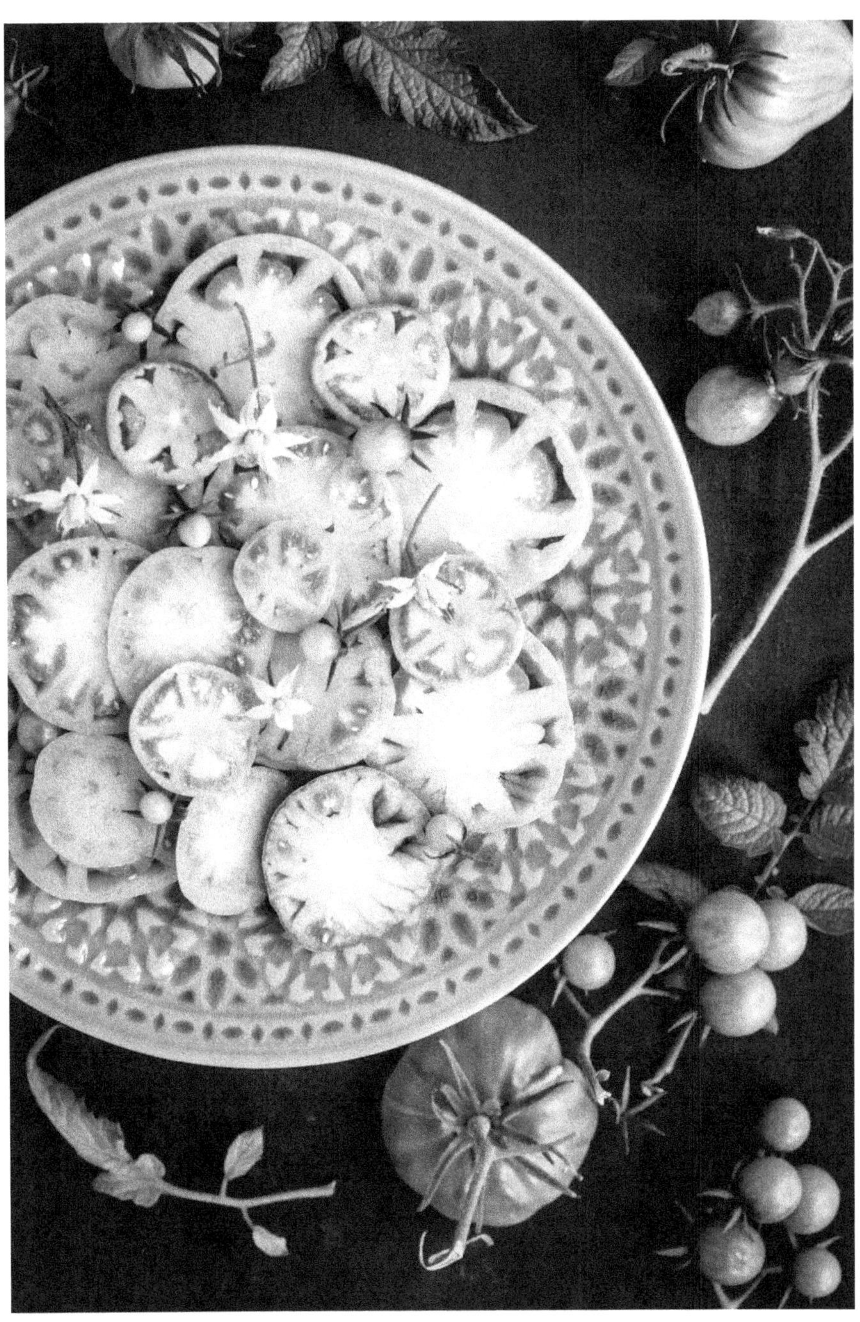

TABLE OF CONTENTS

CONCLUSION 130

INTRODUCTION

Prediabetes – a term that might sound unfamiliar yet carries significant weight for your future health. Imagine your blood sugar levels as a tightrope – normal on one side, full-blown diabetes on the other. Prediabetes is like teetering precariously close to the diabetic side. The good news? You have the power to regain your balance.

The Lowdown on Prediabetes and Its Health Impact:

Prediabetes indicates higher-than-normal blood sugar levels, but not high enough for a diabetes diagnosis. If left unaddressed, it significantly increases your risk of developing type 2 diabetes. Diabetes, in turn, can wreak havoc on your health, potentially leading to heart disease, nerve damage, vision problems, and even kidney failure.

Diet as Your Prediabetes Powerhouse:

The food you choose becomes your weapon against prediabetes. Here's how a strategic diet can help:

- **Blood Sugar Balance:** Certain foods cause blood sugar spikes. Refined carbohydrates like white bread, sugary drinks, and processed snacks are culprits. A prediabetes diet focuses on whole, unprocessed foods like vegetables, fruits, whole grains, and lean protein. These provide sustained energy, preventing those blood sugar rollercoasters.

- **Weight Management**: Often, prediabetes comes hand-in-hand with excess weight. Losing even a modest 5-10% of body weight can significantly improve blood sugar control. A healthy diet naturally promotes weight loss by keeping you feeling fuller for longer and reducing cravings for sugary treats.

The Vegetarian Advantage:

Vegetarian diets, rich in fruits, vegetables, legumes, and whole grains, are a natural fit for prediabetes management. Here's why:

- **Fiber Powerhouse:** Vegetarian meals are bursting with fiber, a magic ingredient that slows down sugar absorption, keeping blood sugar levels stable.

- **Weight Management Ally:** Plant-based diets tend to be lower in calories and fat, making weight loss and management easier. Studies even suggest vegetarians have a lower risk of developing type 2 diabetes overall.

Key Nutritional Principles for Prediabetes Champions:

- **Fiber First:** Aim for at least 25-35 grams of fiber daily. Load up on vegetables, fruits, lentils, beans, and whole grains.
- **Healthy Fats:** Don't fear all fats. Include good fats like those found in nuts, seeds, avocado, and olive oil in your diet.
- **Portion Patrol:** Practice mindful eating. Use smaller plates, chew slowly, and savor your food. This helps you feel satisfied without overeating.
- **Sugar Savvy:** Limit added sugars and refined carbohydrates. Read food labels carefully and choose options with minimal sugar content.

Remember, prediabetes is not a life sentence. By taking charge of your diet and embracing healthy lifestyle choices, you can regain control and significantly reduce your risk of developing diabetes. With dedication and the right dietary tools, you can navigate prediabetes and live a long, healthy life.

Chapter 1: 30 Day Meal Plan

Week 1:

Day 1

- Breakfast: Spinach and Mushroom Tofu Scramble
- Lunch: Lentil and Veggie Buddha Bowl
- Dinner: Eggplant and Chickpea Stew
- Snack: Hummus and Veggie Platter
- Dessert: Berry Chia Seed Pudding

Day 2

- Breakfast: Overnight Chia Seed Pudding
- Lunch: Chickpea Salad with Lemon-Tahini Dressing
- Dinner: Cauliflower "Steak" with Chimichurri Sauce
- Snack: Spicy Roasted Chickpeas
- Dessert: Baked Apple with Cinnamon and Walnuts

Day 3

- Breakfast: Avocado Toast with Tomato and Basil
- Lunch: Quinoa and Black Bean Stuffed Peppers
- Dinner: Stuffed Zucchini Boats with Quinoa
- Snack: Avocado and Black Bean Salsa
- Dessert: Dark Chocolate Avocado Mousse

Day 4

- Breakfast: Quinoa Breakfast Bowl with Berries
- Lunch: Mediterranean Vegetable Wrap
- Dinner: Spinach and Ricotta Stuffed Shells
- Snack: Greek Yogurt with Berries and Honey
- Dessert: Coconut Mango Chia Pudding

Day 5

- Breakfast: Greek Yogurt Parfait with Nuts and Seeds
- Lunch: Spinach and Feta Stuffed Portobello Mushrooms
- Dinner: Vegetable Stir-Fry with Tofu
- Snack: Mini Caprese Skewers
- Dessert: Grilled Peaches with Honey and Yogurt

Day 6

- Breakfast: Oatmeal with Almond Butter and Banana
- Lunch: Roasted Vegetable and Hummus Sandwich
- Dinner: Baked Ratatouille
- Snack: Edamame with Sea Salt
- Dessert: Vegan Chocolate Chip Cookies

Day 7

- Breakfast: Veggie-Packed Breakfast Burrito
- Lunch: Broccoli and Cauliflower Rice Stir-Fry

- Dinner: Spaghetti Squash with Tomato Basil Sauce
- Snack: Almond Butter Stuffed Dates
- Dessert: Banana Nice Cream

Week 2:

Day 8

- Breakfast: Apple-Cinnamon Overnight Oats
- Lunch: Marinated Tofu and Vegetable Skewers
- Dinner: Portobello Mushroom Burgers
- Snack: Baked Zucchini Fries
- Dessert: Almond Butter Brownies

Day 9

- Breakfast: Sweet Potato Hash with Kale
- Lunch: Sweet Potato and Black Bean Tacos
- Dinner: Lentil and Spinach Curry
- Snack: Guacamole with Carrot and Celery Sticks
- Dessert: Chilled Coconut Rice Pudding

Day 10

- Breakfast: Cottage Cheese with Fresh Fruit
- Lunch: Mixed Green Salad with Avocado and Walnuts
- Dinner: Vegan Shepherd's Pie with Lentils

- Snack: Fresh Fruit and Nut Mix

- Dessert: Fresh Berry Salad with Mint

Day 11

- Breakfast: Blueberry and Flaxseed Smoothie Bowl

- Lunch: Thai-Inspired Peanut Noodle Salad

- Dinner: Butternut Squash and Sage Risotto

- Snack: Cottage Cheese and Pineapple Bites

- Dessert: Apple and Oat Crumble

Day 12

- Breakfast: Savory Chickpea Pancakes

- Lunch: Edamame and Quinoa Salad

- Dinner: Grilled Vegetable and Polenta Stack

- Snack: Spinach and Artichoke Dip with Whole Grain Crackers

- Dessert: Pumpkin Spice Energy Balls

Day 13

- Breakfast: Multigrain Porridge with Mixed Nuts

- Lunch: Curried Lentil Soup

- Dinner: Vegan Mushroom Stroganoff

- Snack: Cucumber and Hummus Roll-Ups

- Dessert: Raw Cashew Cheesecake Bites

Day 14

- Breakfast: Zucchini Bread Muffins
- Lunch: Grilled Veggie and Pesto Panini
- Dinner: Sweet Potato and Lentil Dal
- Snack: Tomato Basil Bruschetta
- Dessert: Lemon Blueberry Bars

Week 3:

Day 15

- Breakfast: Tomato and Avocado Breakfast Salad
- Lunch: Kale and Farro Salad with Lemon Vinaigrette
- Dinner: Baked Eggplant Parmesan
- Snack: Mixed Nuts and Seeds Trail Mix
- Dessert: Chocolate Dipped Strawberries

Day 16

- Breakfast: Spinach and Mushroom Tofu Scramble
- Lunch: Lentil and Veggie Buddha Bowl
- Dinner: Eggplant and Chickpea Stew
- Snack: Hummus and Veggie Platter
- Dessert: Berry Chia Seed Pudding

Day 17

- Breakfast: Overnight Chia Seed Pudding
- Lunch: Chickpea Salad with Lemon-Tahini Dressing
- Dinner: Cauliflower "Steak" with Chimichurri Sauce
- Snack: Spicy Roasted Chickpeas
- Dessert: Baked Apple with Cinnamon and Walnuts

Day 18

- Breakfast: Avocado Toast with Tomato and Basil
- Lunch: Quinoa and Black Bean Stuffed Peppers
- Dinner: Stuffed Zucchini Boats with Quinoa
- Snack: Avocado and Black Bean Salsa
- Dessert: Dark Chocolate Avocado Mousse

Day 19

- Breakfast: Quinoa Breakfast Bowl with Berries
- Lunch: Mediterranean Vegetable Wrap
- Dinner: Spinach and Ricotta Stuffed Shells
- Snack: Greek Yogurt with Berries and Honey
- Dessert: Coconut Mango Chia Pudding

Day 20

- Breakfast: Greek Yogurt Parfait with Nuts and Seeds
- Lunch: Spinach and Feta Stuffed Portobello Mushrooms

- Dinner: Vegetable Stir-Fry with Tofu
- Snack: Mini Caprese Skewers
- Dessert: Grilled Peaches with Honey and Yogurt

Day 21

- Breakfast: Oatmeal with Almond Butter and Banana
- Lunch: Roasted Vegetable and Hummus Sandwich
- Dinner: Baked Ratatouille
- Snack: Edamame with Sea Salt
- Dessert: Vegan Chocolate Chip Cookies

Week 4:

Day 22

- Breakfast: Veggie-Packed Breakfast Burrito
- Lunch: Broccoli and Cauliflower Rice Stir-Fry
- Dinner: Spaghetti Squash with Tomato Basil Sauce
- Snack: Almond Butter Stuffed Dates
- Dessert: Banana Nice Cream

Day 23

- Breakfast: Apple-Cinnamon Overnight Oats
- Lunch: Marinated Tofu and Vegetable Skewers
- Dinner: Portobello Mushroom Burgers

- Snack: Baked Zucchini Fries
- Dessert: Almond Butter Brownies

Day 24

- Breakfast: Sweet Potato Hash with Kale
- Lunch: Sweet Potato and Black Bean Tacos
- Dinner: Lentil and Spinach Curry
- Snack: Guacamole with Carrot and Celery Sticks
- Dessert: Chilled Coconut Rice Pudding

Day 25

- Breakfast: Cottage Cheese with Fresh Fruit
- Lunch: Mixed Green Salad with Avocado and Walnuts
- Dinner: Vegan Shepherd's Pie with Lentils
- Snack: Fresh Fruit and Nut Mix
- Dessert: Fresh Berry Salad with Mint

Day 26

- Breakfast: Blueberry and Flaxseed Smoothie Bowl
- Lunch: Thai-Inspired Peanut Noodle Salad
- Dinner: Butternut Squash and Sage Risotto
- Snack: Cottage Cheese and Pineapple Bites
- Dessert: Apple and Oat Crumble

Day 27

- Breakfast: Savory Chickpea Pancakes
- Lunch: Edamame and Quinoa Salad
- Dinner: Grilled Vegetable and Polenta Stack
- Snack: Spinach and Artichoke Dip with Whole Grain Crackers
- Dessert: Pumpkin Spice Energy Balls

Day 28

- Breakfast: Multigrain Porridge with Mixed Nuts
- Lunch: Curried Lentil Soup
- Dinner: Vegan Mushroom Stroganoff
- Snack: Cucumber and Hummus Roll-Ups
- Dessert: Raw Cashew Cheesecake Bites

Day 29

- Breakfast: Zucchini Bread Muffins
- Lunch: Grilled Veggie and Pesto Panini
- Dinner: Sweet Potato and Lentil Dal
- Snack: Tomato Basil Bruschetta
- Dessert: Lemon Blueberry Bars

Day 30

- Breakfast: Tomato and Avocado Breakfast Salad

- Lunch: Kale and Farro Salad with Lemon Vinaigrette

- Dinner: Baked Eggplant Parmesan

- Snack: Mixed Nuts and Seeds Trail Mix

- Dessert: Chocolate Dipped Strawberries

Chapter 2: Breakfast Recipes

Starting your day with a nutritious and satisfying breakfast can make a significant difference in managing prediabetes and promoting weight loss. The following vegetarian recipes are designed to provide a balance of proteins, healthy fats, and complex carbohydrates to keep you energized and satisfied throughout the morning.

Spinach and Mushroom Tofu Scramble

Ingredients:

- 1 block firm tofu, crumbled
- 1 cup spinach, chopped
- 1 cup mushrooms, sliced
- 1 small onion, diced
- 1 clove garlic, minced
- 1 tablespoon olive oil
- 1 teaspoon turmeric
- Salt and pepper to taste

Instructions:

1. Heat olive oil in a pan over medium heat.
2. Sauté onions and garlic until translucent.

3. Add mushrooms and cook until tender.

4. Stir in crumbled tofu, turmeric, salt, and pepper.

5. Cook for 5 minutes, then add spinach.

6. Cook until spinach is wilted.

Nutrition Information (per serving):

- Calories: 180
- Protein: 15g
- Carbohydrates: 8g
- Fat: 10g
- Fiber: 3g
- Sugar: 2g
- Portion Size: 1 cup

Overnight Chia Seed Pudding

Ingredients:

- 1/4 cup chia seeds
- 1 cup almond milk
- 1 tablespoon maple syrup
- 1/2 teaspoon vanilla extract
- Fresh berries for topping

Instructions:

1. Mix chia seeds, almond milk, maple syrup, and vanilla extract in a jar.
2. Stir well, cover, and refrigerate overnight.
3. Top with fresh berries before serving.

Nutrition Information (per serving):

- Calories: 200
- Protein: 5g
- Carbohydrates: 24g
- Fat: 10g
- Fiber: 10g
- Sugar: 10g
- Portion Size: 1 cup

Avocado Toast with Tomato and Basil

Ingredients:

- 1 slice whole grain bread, toasted
- 1/2 avocado, mashed
- 1 small tomato, sliced
- Fresh basil leaves
- Salt and pepper to taste

Instructions:

1. Spread mashed avocado on toast.

2. Top with tomato slices and basil leaves.

3. Season with salt and pepper.

Nutrition Information (per serving):

- Calories: 250

- Protein: 6g

- Carbohydrates: 30g

- Fat: 15g

- Fiber: 8g

- Sugar: 3g

- Portion Size: 1 slice

Quinoa Breakfast Bowl with Berries

Ingredients:

- 1 cup cooked quinoa

- 1/2 cup mixed berries

- 1 tablespoon almond butter

- 1 tablespoon chia seeds

- 1 teaspoon honey

Instructions:

1. Place cooked quinoa in a bowl.
2. Top with berries, almond butter, chia seeds, and honey.

Nutrition Information (per serving):

- Calories: 320
- Protein: 9g
- Carbohydrates: 50g
- Fat: 10g
- Fiber: 9g
- Sugar: 15g
- Portion Size: 1 bowl

Greek Yogurt Parfait with Nuts and Seeds

Ingredients:

- 1 cup Greek yogurt
- 1/4 cup mixed nuts and seeds
- 1 tablespoon honey
- Fresh fruit for topping

Instructions:

1. Layer Greek yogurt in a bowl.

2. Top with mixed nuts, seeds, honey, and fresh fruit.

Nutrition Information (per serving):

- Calories: 300
- Protein: 15g
- Carbohydrates: 35g
- Fat: 12g
- Fiber: 4g
- Sugar: 25g
- Portion Size: 1 cup

Oatmeal with Almond Butter and Banana

Ingredients:

- 1/2 cup rolled oats
- 1 cup water or milk
- 1 tablespoon almond butter
- 1 banana, sliced
- 1 teaspoon cinnamon

Instructions:

1. Cook oats in water or milk according to package instructions.

2. Stir in almond butter and top with banana slices and cinnamon.

Nutrition Information (per serving):

- Calories: 350
- Protein: 8g
- Carbohydrates: 55g
- Fat: 12g
- Fiber: 8g
- Sugar: 15g
- Portion Size: 1 bowl

Veggie-Packed Breakfast Burrito

Ingredients:

- 1 whole wheat tortilla
- 1/4 cup black beans, cooked
- 1/4 cup corn kernels
- 1/4 cup diced bell peppers
- 1/4 cup spinach, chopped
- 1 tablespoon salsa
- 1 tablespoon shredded cheese

Instructions:

1. Warm the tortilla in a pan.

2. Fill with black beans, corn, bell peppers, spinach, salsa, and cheese.

3. Roll up and serve warm.

Nutrition Information (per serving):

- Calories: 320

- Protein: 12g

- Carbohydrates: 45g

- Fat: 10g

- Fiber: 10g

- Sugar: 5g

- Portion Size: 1 burrito

Apple-Cinnamon Overnight Oats

Ingredients:

- 1/2 cup rolled oats

- 1/2 cup almond milk

- 1/2 apple, diced

- 1 teaspoon cinnamon

- 1 tablespoon chia seeds

Instructions:

1. Mix oats, almond milk, apple, cinnamon, and chia seeds in a jar.
2. Stir well, cover, and refrigerate overnight.

Nutrition Information (per serving):

- Calories: 250
- Protein: 6g
- Carbohydrates: 40g
- Fat: 8g
- Fiber: 8g
- Sugar: 10g
- Portion Size: 1 cup

Sweet Potato Hash with Kale

Ingredients:

- 1 medium sweet potato, diced
- 1 cup kale, chopped
- 1 small onion, diced
- 1 tablespoon olive oil
- Salt and pepper to taste

Instructions:

1. Heat olive oil in a pan over medium heat.
2. Sauté onions until translucent.
3. Add sweet potatoes and cook until tender.
4. Stir in kale and cook until wilted.
5. Season with salt and pepper.

Nutrition Information (per serving):

- Calories: 200
- Protein: 3g
- Carbohydrates: 35g
- Fat: 8g
- Fiber: 6g
- Sugar: 8g
- Portion Size: 1 cup

Cottage Cheese with Fresh Fruit

Ingredients:

- 1 cup cottage cheese
- 1/2 cup fresh fruit (e.g., berries, pineapple, peach)
- 1 tablespoon honey (optional)

Instructions:

1. Scoop cottage cheese into a bowl.
2. Top with fresh fruit and drizzle with honey if desired.

Nutrition Information (per serving):

- Calories: 200
- Protein: 15g
- Carbohydrates: 20g
- Fat: 5g
- Fiber: 2g
- Sugar: 15g
- Portion Size: 1 cup

Blueberry and Flaxseed Smoothie Bowl

Ingredients:

- 1 cup frozen blueberries
- 1/2 banana
- 1/2 cup Greek yogurt
- 1/4 cup almond milk
- 1 tablespoon flaxseed meal
- Fresh fruit and nuts for topping

Instructions:

1. Blend blueberries, banana, Greek yogurt, almond milk, and flaxseed meal until smooth.

2. Pour into a bowl and top with fresh fruit and nuts.

Nutrition Information (per serving):

- Calories: 250

- Protein: 12g

- Carbohydrates: 40g

- Fat: 8g

- Fiber: 7g

- Sugar: 25g

- Portion Size: 1 bowl

Savory Chickpea Pancakes

Ingredients:

- 1 cup chickpea flour

- 1/2 cup water

- 1/2 cup chopped vegetables (e.g., spinach, tomatoes, onions)

- 1 teaspoon cumin

- Salt and pepper to taste

- Olive oil for cooking

Instructions:

1. Mix chickpea flour and water to form a batter.
2. Stir in chopped vegetables, cumin, salt, and pepper.
3. Heat olive oil in a pan over medium heat.
4. Pour batter into the pan and cook until golden brown on both sides.

Nutrition Information (per serving):

*   Calories: 220
*   Protein: 10g
*   Carbohydrates: 30g
*   Fat: 6g
*   Fiber: 5g
*   Sugar: 4g
*   Portion Size: 2 pancakes

Multigrain Porridge with Mixed Nuts

Ingredients:

*   1/2 cup multigrain cereal
*   1 cup water or milk
*   1/4 cup mixed nuts
*   1 tablespoon honey

Instructions:

1. Cook multigrain cereal in water or milk according to package instructions.
2. Top with mixed nuts and honey before serving.

Nutrition Information (per serving):

- Calories: 300
- Protein: 8g
- Carbohydrates: 45g
- Fat: 12g
- Fiber: 6g
- Sugar: 15g
- Portion Size: 1 bowl

Zucchini Bread Muffins

Ingredients:

- 1 cup grated zucchini
- 1 cup whole wheat flour
- 1/2 cup almond flour
- 1/2 cup honey
- 1/4 cup olive oil
- 2 eggs
- 1 teaspoon baking powder

- 1 teaspoon cinnamon

Instructions:

1. Preheat oven to 350°F (175°C).
2. Mix all ingredients in a bowl until well combined.
3. Pour batter into muffin tins.
4. Bake for 20-25 minutes or until a toothpick comes out clean.

Nutrition Information (per serving):

- Calories: 180
- Protein: 4g
- Carbohydrates: 25g
- Fat: 8g
- Fiber: 3g
- Sugar: 12g
- Portion Size: 1 muffin

Tomato and Avocado Breakfast Salad

Ingredients:

- 1 avocado, diced
- 2 tomatoes, chopped
- 1/4 cup red onion, diced
- 1 tablespoon olive oil

- 1 tablespoon lemon juice
- Salt and pepper to taste

Instructions:

1. Combine avocado, tomatoes, and red onion in a bowl.
2. Drizzle with olive oil and lemon juice.
3. Season with salt and pepper and toss gently.

Nutrition Information (per serving):

- Calories: 220
- Protein: 3g
- Carbohydrates: 15g
- Fat: 18g
- Fiber: 7g
- Sugar: 5g
- Portion Size: 1 bowl

Chapter 3: Lunch Recipes

This chapter presents a variety of vegetarian lunch recipes designed to be both delicious and healthy. Each recipe focuses on nutrient-dense ingredients, offering a balance of proteins, healthy fats, and complex carbohydrates. Enjoy these flavorful dishes that are perfect for weight loss and blood sugar control.

Lentil and Veggie Buddha Bowl

Ingredients:

- 1 cup cooked lentils
- 1 cup quinoa, cooked
- 1 cup steamed broccoli
- 1 cup roasted sweet potatoes, cubed
- 1/2 avocado, sliced
- 1/4 cup shredded carrots
- 2 tbsp tahini
- 1 tbsp lemon juice
- 1 tbsp olive oil
- Salt and pepper to taste

Instructions:

1. Combine tahini, lemon juice, olive oil, salt, and pepper to make the dressing.
2. Arrange lentils, quinoa, broccoli, sweet potatoes, avocado, and carrots in a bowl.
3. Drizzle with dressing and serve.

Nutrition Information:

- Calories: 520
- Protein: 18g
- Carbohydrates: 67g
- Fat: 21g
- Fiber: 15g
- Sugar: 6g
- Portion size: 1 bowl

Chickpea Salad with Lemon-Tahini Dressing

Ingredients:

- 1 can chickpeas, drained and rinsed
- 1/2 cucumber, diced
- 1/2 red bell pepper, diced
- 1/4 red onion, finely chopped

- 2 tbsp fresh parsley, chopped
- 2 tbsp tahini
- 1 tbsp lemon juice
- 1 tbsp olive oil
- Salt and pepper to taste

Instructions:

1. In a bowl, mix chickpeas, cucumber, red bell pepper, red onion, and parsley.
2. In a separate bowl, whisk tahini, lemon juice, olive oil, salt, and pepper.
3. Pour dressing over chickpea mixture and toss to combine.

Nutrition Information:

- Calories: 320
- Protein: 10g
- Carbohydrates: 34g
- Fat: 18g
- Fiber: 8g
- Sugar: 5g
- Portion size: 1 bowl

Quinoa and Black Bean Stuffed Peppers

Ingredients:

- 4 bell peppers, tops removed and seeds scooped out
- 1 cup cooked quinoa
- 1 can black beans, drained and rinsed
- 1 cup corn kernels
- 1/2 cup diced tomatoes
- 1 tsp cumin
- 1 tsp chili powder
- Salt and pepper to taste
- 1/4 cup shredded cheese (optional)

Instructions:

1. Preheat oven to 375°F (190°C).
2. In a bowl, mix quinoa, black beans, corn, tomatoes, cumin, chili powder, salt, and pepper.
3. Stuff bell peppers with the mixture and place them in a baking dish.
4. Top with cheese if using and bake for 25-30 minutes.

Nutrition Information:

- Calories: 260
- Protein: 10g
- Carbohydrates: 45g

- Fat: 5g

- Fiber: 11g

- Sugar: 8g

- Portion size: 1 stuffed pepper

Mediterranean Vegetable Wrap

Ingredients:

- 1 whole wheat tortilla

- 1/2 cup hummus

- 1/2 cup spinach leaves

- 1/4 cup cucumber slices

- 1/4 cup roasted red peppers

- 2 tbsp feta cheese, crumbled

- 1 tbsp olives, sliced

Instructions:

1. Spread hummus evenly over the tortilla.

2. Layer spinach, cucumber, roasted red peppers, feta cheese, and olives.

3. Roll up the tortilla tightly and slice in half.

Nutrition Information:

- Calories: 350

- Protein: 10g

- Carbohydrates: 45g

- Fat: 15g

- Fiber: 8g

- Sugar: 4g

- Portion size: 1 wrap

Spinach and Feta Stuffed Portobello Mushrooms

Ingredients:

- 4 large Portobello mushrooms, stems removed

- 1 cup fresh spinach, chopped

- 1/2 cup feta cheese, crumbled

- 2 cloves garlic, minced

- 1 tbsp olive oil

- Salt and pepper to taste

Instructions:

1. Preheat oven to 375°F (190°C).

2. In a bowl, mix spinach, feta cheese, garlic, olive oil, salt, and pepper.

3. Stuff mushrooms with the mixture and place on a baking sheet.

4. Bake for 20-25 minutes.

Nutrition Information:

- Calories: 150
- Protein: 7g
- Carbohydrates: 8g
- Fat: 10g
- Fiber: 3g
- Sugar: 3g
- Portion size: 1 mushroom

Roasted Vegetable and Hummus Sandwich

Ingredients:

- 2 slices whole grain bread
- 1/2 cup mixed roasted vegetables (zucchini, bell peppers, eggplant)
- 1/4 cup hummus
- 1 handful arugula
- Salt and pepper to taste

Instructions:

1. Spread hummus on both slices of bread.

2. Layer roasted vegetables and arugula on one slice.

3. Top with the second slice and cut in half.

Nutrition Information:

- Calories: 350
- Protein: 10g
- Carbohydrates: 50g
- Fat: 12g
- Fiber: 9g
- Sugar: 6g
- Portion size: 1 sandwich

Broccoli and Cauliflower Rice Stir-Fry

Ingredients:

- 1 cup broccoli florets
- 1 cup cauliflower rice
- 1/2 bell pepper, sliced
- 1 carrot, julienned
- 2 tbsp soy sauce
- 1 tbsp sesame oil
- 1 clove garlic, minced
- 1 tsp ginger, grated

Instructions:

1. Heat sesame oil in a pan over medium heat.

2. Add garlic and ginger, sauté for 1 minute.

3. Add broccoli, bell pepper, and carrot, cook for 5 minutes.

4. Stir in cauliflower rice and soy sauce, cook for another 3 minutes.

Nutrition Information:

- Calories: 180

- Protein: 6g

- Carbohydrates: 20g

- Fat: 9g

- Fiber: 6g

- Sugar: 6g

- Portion size: 1 bowl

Marinated Tofu and Vegetable Skewers

Ingredients:

- 1 block firm tofu, cubed

- 1 zucchini, sliced

- 1 bell pepper, chopped

- 1 red onion, chopped

- 1/4 cup soy sauce

- 2 tbsp olive oil
- 1 tbsp lemon juice
- 1 tsp garlic powder
- 1 tsp paprika

Instructions:

1. Mix soy sauce, olive oil, lemon juice, garlic powder, and paprika to make the marinade.
2. Marinate tofu and vegetables for at least 30 minutes.
3. Thread tofu and vegetables onto skewers.
4. Grill or bake at 375°F (190°C) for 20 minutes, turning occasionally.

Nutrition Information:

- Calories: 250
- Protein: 12g
- Carbohydrates: 15g
- Fat: 16g
- Fiber: 4g
- Sugar: 5g
- Portion size: 2 skewers

Sweet Potato and Black Bean Tacos

Ingredients:

- 1 large sweet potato, diced
- 1 can black beans, drained and rinsed
- 1 avocado, sliced
- 1/4 cup red onion, diced
- 1/4 cup cilantro, chopped
- 1 tsp cumin
- 1 tsp chili powder
- Salt and pepper to taste
- 4 small corn tortillas

Instructions:

1. Preheat oven to 400°F (200°C).
2. Toss sweet potato with cumin, chili powder, salt, and pepper. Roast for 20-25 minutes.
3. Warm tortillas and fill with sweet potato, black beans, avocado, red onion, and cilantro.

Nutrition Information:

- Calories: 320
- Protein: 9g
- Carbohydrates: 50g
- Fat: 10g

- Fiber: 12g
- Sugar: 6g
- Portion size: 2 tacos

Mixed Green Salad with Avocado and Walnuts

Ingredients:

- 4 cups mixed greens
- 1 avocado, sliced
- 1/4 cup walnuts, chopped
- 1/4 cup cherry tomatoes, halved
- 1/4 red onion, thinly sliced
- 2 tbsp balsamic vinaigrette

Instructions:

1. In a large bowl, combine mixed greens, avocado, walnuts, cherry tomatoes, and red onion.
2. Drizzle with balsamic vinaigrette and toss gently.

Nutrition Information:

- Calories: 300
- Protein: 5g
- Carbohydrates: 20g

- Fat: 26g

- Fiber: 9g

- Sugar: 6g

- Portion size: 1 bowl

Thai-Inspired Peanut Noodle Salad

Ingredients:

- 4 oz rice noodles, cooked

- 1/2 cup shredded carrots

- 1/2 cup red bell pepper, sliced

- 1/4 cup green onions, chopped

- 2 tbsp cilantro, chopped

- 1/4 cup peanut butter

- 2 tbsp soy sauce

- 1 tbsp lime juice

- 1 tsp ginger, grated

- 1 tsp honey

Instructions:

1. Whisk peanut butter, soy sauce, lime juice, ginger, and honey to make the dressing.

2. Toss cooked noodles with carrots, bell pepper, green onions, and cilantro.

3. Pour dressing over noodle mixture and toss to combine.

Nutrition Information:

- Calories: 350
- Protein: 10g
- Carbohydrates: 55g
- Fat: 12g
- Fiber: 5g
- Sugar: 8g
- Portion size: 1 bowl

Edamame and Quinoa Salad

Ingredients:

- 1 cup cooked quinoa
- 1 cup shelled edamame
- 1/2 cup diced cucumber
- 1/2 cup diced red bell pepper
- 2 tbsp green onions, chopped
- 2 tbsp rice vinegar
- 1 tbsp sesame oil
- 1 tsp soy sauce
- Salt and pepper to taste

Instructions:

1. In a large bowl, combine quinoa, edamame, cucumber, bell pepper, and green onions.

2. In a small bowl, whisk rice vinegar, sesame oil, soy sauce, salt, and pepper.

3. Pour dressing over quinoa mixture and toss to combine.

Nutrition Information:

- Calories: 260
- Protein: 10g
- Carbohydrates: 35g
- Fat: 9g
- Fiber: 6g
- Sugar: 4g
- Portion size: 1 bowl

Curried Lentil Soup

Ingredients:

- 1 cup red lentils, rinsed
- 1 carrot, diced
- 1 celery stalk, diced
- 1 small onion, chopped
- 2 cloves garlic, minced

- 1 tbsp curry powder
- 1 tsp turmeric
- 4 cups vegetable broth
- 1 can coconut milk
- Salt and pepper to taste

Instructions:

1. In a large pot, sauté onion, garlic, carrot, and celery until soft.
2. Add curry powder and turmeric, cook for 1 minute.
3. Stir in lentils, vegetable broth, and coconut milk. Bring to a boil.
4. Reduce heat and simmer for 20-25 minutes until lentils are tender.

Nutrition Information:

- Calories: 350
- Protein: 14g
- Carbohydrates: 45g
- Fat: 14g
- Fiber: 12g
- Sugar: 5g
- Portion size: 1 bowl

Grilled Veggie and Pesto Panini

Ingredients:

- 2 slices whole grain bread
- 1/4 cup pesto
- 1/2 cup grilled zucchini slices
- 1/2 cup grilled red bell pepper
- 1/4 cup mozzarella cheese, shredded

Instructions:

1. Spread pesto on both slices of bread.
2. Layer grilled zucchini, bell pepper, and mozzarella cheese.
3. Press sandwich in a panini maker until bread is toasted and cheese is melted.

Nutrition Information:

- Calories: 400
- Protein: 14g
- Carbohydrates: 45g
- Fat: 18g
- Fiber: 7g
- Sugar: 4g
- Portion size: 1 panini

Kale and Farro Salad with Lemon Vinaigrette

Ingredients:

- 2 cups kale, chopped
- 1 cup cooked farro
- 1/4 cup dried cranberries
- 1/4 cup walnuts, chopped
- 1/4 cup feta cheese, crumbled
- 2 tbsp olive oil
- 1 tbsp lemon juice
- 1 tsp Dijon mustard
- Salt and pepper to taste

Instructions:

1. In a large bowl, combine kale, farro, cranberries, walnuts, and feta cheese.
2. In a small bowl, whisk olive oil, lemon juice, Dijon mustard, salt, and pepper.
3. Pour dressing over salad and toss to combine.

Nutrition Information:

- Calories: 300
- Protein: 10g
- Carbohydrates: 35g

- Fat: 15g
- Fiber: 8g
- Sugar: 7g
- Portion size: 1 bowl

Chapter 4: Dinner Recipes

Managing prediabetes doesn't mean sacrificing taste or satisfaction at dinner. These vegetarian recipes are crafted to offer delicious and nutrient-rich meals that support weight loss and blood sugar management. Each recipe is designed to provide a balanced mix of proteins, healthy fats, and complex carbohydrates, ensuring you stay full and energized.

Eggplant and Chickpea Stew

Ingredients:

- 1 large eggplant, diced
- 1 can chickpeas, drained and rinsed
- 1 onion, chopped
- 2 garlic cloves, minced
- 1 can diced tomatoes
- 2 cups vegetable broth
- 1 tsp cumin
- 1 tsp paprika
- Salt and pepper to taste
- 2 tbsp olive oil
- Fresh parsley for garnish

Instructions:

1. Heat olive oil in a pot over medium heat. Add onion and garlic, and sauté until softened.
2. Add diced eggplant and cook until it begins to soften.
3. Stir in chickpeas, diced tomatoes, vegetable broth, cumin, paprika, salt, and pepper.
4. Bring to a boil, then reduce heat and simmer for 25-30 minutes, until the eggplant is tender.
5. Garnish with fresh parsley before serving.

Nutrition Information (per serving):

- Calories: 220
- Protein: 6g
- Carbohydrates: 28g
- Fat: 10g
- Fiber: 9g
- Sugar: 8g
- Portion Size: 1 cup

Cauliflower "Steak" with Chimichurri Sauce

Ingredients:

- 1 large cauliflower head, cut into 1-inch steaks

- 2 tbsp olive oil
- Salt and pepper to taste
- 1 cup fresh parsley
- 1/2 cup olive oil
- 2 tbsp red wine vinegar
- 3 garlic cloves
- 1 tsp red pepper flakes
- Salt and pepper to taste

Instructions:

1. Preheat oven to 400°F (200°C).
2. Brush cauliflower steaks with olive oil, season with salt and pepper, and place on a baking sheet.
3. Roast for 25-30 minutes, flipping halfway through, until golden brown.
4. For the chimichurri sauce, blend parsley, olive oil, vinegar, garlic, red pepper flakes, salt, and pepper until smooth.
5. Drizzle the chimichurri sauce over the roasted cauliflower steaks before serving.

Nutrition Information (per serving):

- Calories: 180
- Protein: 2g
- Carbohydrates: 8g

- Fat: 16g

- Fiber: 4g

- Sugar: 2g

- Portion Size: 1 steak with sauce

Stuffed Zucchini Boats with Quinoa

Ingredients:

- 4 large zucchinis, halved lengthwise and seeds scooped out

- 1 cup cooked quinoa

- 1 can black beans, drained and rinsed

- 1 cup corn kernels

- 1 bell pepper, diced

- 1 onion, chopped

- 2 garlic cloves, minced

- 1 tsp cumin

- 1 tsp chili powder

- Salt and pepper to taste

- 1/2 cup shredded cheese (optional)

- 2 tbsp olive oil

Instructions:

1. Preheat oven to 375°F (190°C).

2. Heat olive oil in a pan over medium heat. Sauté onion and garlic until softened.

3. Add bell pepper, corn, black beans, cooked quinoa, cumin, chili powder, salt, and pepper. Cook for 5 minutes.

4. Fill zucchini halves with the mixture and place them in a baking dish.

5. Top with shredded cheese if using.

6. Bake for 25-30 minutes until zucchini is tender and cheese is melted.

Nutrition Information (per serving):

- Calories: 240
- Protein: 9g
- Carbohydrates: 35g
- Fat: 8g
- Fiber: 10g
- Sugar: 6g
- Portion Size: 1 stuffed zucchini half

Spinach and Ricotta Stuffed Shells

Ingredients:

- 20 jumbo pasta shells
- 2 cups ricotta cheese

- 1 cup shredded mozzarella cheese
- 1/2 cup grated Parmesan cheese
- 2 cups fresh spinach, chopped
- 1 egg, beaten
- 2 cups marinara sauce
- Salt and pepper to taste

Instructions:

1. Preheat oven to 375°F (190°C). Cook pasta shells according to package instructions.
2. In a bowl, mix ricotta, 1/2 cup mozzarella, Parmesan, spinach, egg, salt, and pepper.
3. Fill each pasta shell with the ricotta mixture.
4. Spread 1 cup of marinara sauce on the bottom of a baking dish. Place stuffed shells in the dish and top with remaining marinara sauce and mozzarella cheese.
5. Cover with foil and bake for 25 minutes. Remove foil and bake for an additional 10 minutes until cheese is bubbly.

Nutrition Information (per serving):

- Calories: 320
- Protein: 18g
- Carbohydrates: 28g
- Fat: 15g

- Fiber: 4g

- Sugar: 6g

- Portion Size: 4 stuffed shells

Vegetable Stir-Fry with Tofu

Ingredients:

- 1 block firm tofu, cubed

- 1 cup broccoli florets

- 1 bell pepper, sliced

- 1 carrot, sliced

- 1 onion, sliced

- 2 garlic cloves, minced

- 2 tbsp soy sauce

- 1 tbsp sesame oil

- 1 tbsp olive oil

- 1 tsp cornstarch mixed with 2 tbsp water

- Salt and pepper to taste

- Cooked brown rice for serving

Instructions:

1. Heat olive oil in a large pan over medium-high heat. Add tofu and cook until golden brown, then set aside.

2. In the same pan, add sesame oil and sauté garlic and onion until fragrant.

3. Add broccoli, bell pepper, and carrot. Stir-fry until vegetables are tender-crisp.

4. Return tofu to the pan, add soy sauce, and cornstarch mixture. Stir well to coat everything in the sauce.

5. Season with salt and pepper to taste and serve over cooked brown rice.

Nutrition Information (per serving):

- Calories: 270
- Protein: 12g
- Carbohydrates: 20g
- Fat: 16g
- Fiber: 5g
- Sugar: 5g
- Portion Size: 1 cup

Baked Ratatouille

Ingredients:

- 1 eggplant, thinly sliced
- 2 zucchinis, thinly sliced
- 1 yellow squash, thinly sliced

- 1 red bell pepper, thinly sliced
- 1 yellow bell pepper, thinly sliced
- 1 onion, thinly sliced
- 3 tomatoes, thinly sliced
- 3 garlic cloves, minced
- 2 cups tomato sauce
- 2 tbsp olive oil
- Fresh thyme and basil for garnish
- Salt and pepper to taste

Instructions:

1. Preheat oven to 375°F (190°C).
2. Spread tomato sauce on the bottom of a baking dish. Layer sliced vegetables in an alternating pattern.
3. Sprinkle minced garlic over the vegetables. Drizzle with olive oil and season with salt and pepper.
4. Cover with foil and bake for 40 minutes. Remove foil and bake for an additional 10 minutes.
5. Garnish with fresh thyme and basil before serving.

Nutrition Information (per serving):

- Calories: 200
- Protein: 4g
- Carbohydrates: 26g

- Fat: 10g

- Fiber: 8g

- Sugar: 12g

- Portion Size: 1 cup

Spaghetti Squash with Tomato Basil Sauce

Ingredients:

- 1 large spaghetti squash

- 2 cups cherry tomatoes, halved

- 3 garlic cloves, minced

- 1/4 cup fresh basil, chopped

- 1/4 cup grated Parmesan cheese

- 2 tbsp olive oil

- Salt and pepper to taste

Instructions:

1. Preheat oven to 400°F (200°C). Cut spaghetti squash in half lengthwise and remove seeds.

2. Drizzle with olive oil, season with salt and pepper, and place cut side down on a baking sheet. Bake for 40 minutes until tender.

3. While the squash bakes, heat olive oil in a pan over medium heat. Sauté garlic until fragrant, then add cherry tomatoes and cook until softened.

4. Use a fork to scrape the spaghetti squash strands into a bowl. Toss with tomato mixture, fresh basil, and Parmesan cheese.

5. Season with salt and pepper before serving.

Nutrition Information (per serving):

- Calories: 180
- Protein: 4g
- Carbohydrates: 22g
- Fat: 9g
- Fiber: 5g
- Sugar: 8g
- Portion Size: 1 cup

Portobello Mushroom Burgers

Ingredients:

- 4 large portobello mushrooms, stems removed
- 2 tbsp balsamic vinegar
- 2 tbsp olive oil
- 1 tsp garlic powder
- 1 tsp onion powder

- Salt and pepper to taste
- 4 whole grain buns
- Lettuce, tomato, and onion slices for serving

Instructions:

1. Preheat grill to medium-high heat.
2. In a bowl, mix balsamic vinegar, olive oil, garlic powder, onion powder, salt, and pepper.
3. Brush portobello mushrooms with the marinade and let sit for 10 minutes.
4. Grill mushrooms for 5-7 minutes per side until tender.
5. Serve on whole grain buns with lettuce, tomato, and onion slices.

Nutrition Information (per serving):

- Calories: 250
- Protein: 6g
- Carbohydrates: 30g
- Fat: 12g
- Fiber: 6g
- Sugar: 5g
- Portion Size: 1 burger

Lentil and Spinach Curry

Ingredients:

- 1 cup green lentils, rinsed
- 2 cups fresh spinach, chopped
- 1 onion, chopped
- 2 garlic cloves, minced
- 1 can coconut milk
- 2 cups vegetable broth
- 1 tbsp curry powder
- 1 tsp cumin
- 1 tsp turmeric
- Salt and pepper to taste
- 2 tbsp olive oil

Instructions:

1. Heat olive oil in a pot over medium heat. Sauté onion and garlic until softened.
2. Add curry powder, cumin, turmeric, salt, and pepper. Cook for 1 minute.
3. Stir in lentils, vegetable broth, and coconut milk. Bring to a boil, then reduce heat and simmer for 25-30 minutes until lentils are tender.
4. Stir in chopped spinach and cook for an additional 5 minutes.
5. Serve hot.

Nutrition Information (per serving):

- Calories: 310
- Protein: 13g
- Carbohydrates: 36g
- Fat: 14g
- Fiber: 12g
- Sugar: 4g
- Portion Size: 1 cup

Vegan Shepherd's Pie with Lentils

Ingredients:

- 2 cups cooked lentils
- 1 onion, chopped
- 2 garlic cloves, minced
- 2 carrots, diced
- 1 cup peas
- 1 cup corn kernels
- 1 cup vegetable broth
- 2 tbsp tomato paste
- 1 tsp thyme
- 1 tsp rosemary
- Salt and pepper to taste
- 4 cups mashed potatoes

- 2 tbsp olive oil

Instructions:

1. Preheat oven to 375°F (190°C).
2. Heat olive oil in a pan over medium heat. Sauté onion and garlic until softened.
3. Add carrots, peas, corn, cooked lentils, vegetable broth, tomato paste, thyme, rosemary, salt, and pepper. Cook for 10 minutes until vegetables are tender.
4. Spread the lentil mixture in a baking dish and top with mashed potatoes.
5. Bake for 20-25 minutes until the top is golden brown.

Nutrition Information (per serving):

- Calories: 350
- Protein: 10g
- Carbohydrates: 52g
- Fat: 12g
- Fiber: 10g
- Sugar: 7g
- Portion Size: 1 cup

Butternut Squash and Sage Risotto

Ingredients:

- 1 cup Arborio rice
- 2 cups butternut squash, cubed
- 1 onion, chopped
- 3 garlic cloves, minced
- 4 cups vegetable broth
- 1/4 cup dry white wine (optional)
- 2 tbsp olive oil
- 1/4 cup grated Parmesan cheese
- 2 tbsp fresh sage, chopped
- Salt and pepper to taste

Instructions:

1. Heat olive oil in a pot over medium heat. Sauté onion and garlic until softened.
2. Add Arborio rice and cook for 2 minutes, stirring constantly.
3. Pour in white wine, if using, and cook until absorbed.
4. Gradually add vegetable broth, 1 cup at a time, stirring constantly until the liquid is absorbed before adding more.
5. When the rice is almost tender, add butternut squash and cook until tender.
6. Stir in Parmesan cheese, fresh sage, salt, and pepper before serving.

Nutrition Information (per serving):

- Calories: 320
- Protein: 7g
- Carbohydrates: 50g
- Fat: 10g
- Fiber: 4g
- Sugar: 4g
- Portion Size: 1 cup

Grilled Vegetable and Polenta Stack

Ingredients:

- 1 tube polenta, sliced into rounds
- 1 eggplant, sliced
- 1 zucchini, sliced
- 1 red bell pepper, sliced
- 1 yellow bell pepper, sliced
- 2 tbsp olive oil
- 1/4 cup balsamic vinegar
- Salt and pepper to taste
- Fresh basil for garnish

Instructions:

1. Preheat grill to medium-high heat.

2. Brush polenta and vegetables with olive oil and season with salt and pepper.

3. Grill polenta rounds for 3-4 minutes per side until golden. Grill vegetables until tender.

4. Stack grilled polenta and vegetables, drizzle with balsamic vinegar, and garnish with fresh basil before serving.

Nutrition Information (per serving):

- Calories: 230
- Protein: 4g
- Carbohydrates: 28g
- Fat: 12g
- Fiber: 6g
- Sugar: 8g
- Portion Size: 1 stack

Vegan Mushroom Stroganoff

Ingredients:

- 1 lb mushrooms, sliced
- 1 onion, chopped
- 2 garlic cloves, minced

- 1 cup vegetable broth
- 1/2 cup coconut milk
- 2 tbsp soy sauce
- 2 tbsp flour
- 2 tbsp olive oil
- 1 tsp paprika
- Salt and pepper to taste
- Cooked whole wheat pasta for serving

Instructions:

1. Heat olive oil in a pan over medium heat. Sauté onion and garlic until softened.
2. Add mushrooms and cook until browned.
3. Sprinkle flour over the mushrooms and stir to coat.
4. Pour in vegetable broth, soy sauce, and coconut milk. Stir until the sauce thickens.
5. Season with paprika, salt, and pepper. Serve over cooked whole wheat pasta.

Nutrition Information (per serving):

- Calories: 280
- Protein: 8g
- Carbohydrates: 30g
- Fat: 14g

- Fiber: 6g

- Sugar: 4g

- Portion Size: 1 cup

Sweet Potato and Lentil Dal

Ingredients:

- 1 cup red lentils, rinsed

- 2 sweet potatoes, peeled and diced

- 1 onion, chopped

- 3 garlic cloves, minced

- 1 tbsp ginger, grated

- 1 can coconut milk

- 3 cups vegetable broth

- 2 tbsp curry powder

- 1 tsp cumin

- Salt and pepper to taste

- 2 tbsp olive oil

Instructions:

1. Heat olive oil in a pot over medium heat. Sauté onion, garlic, and ginger until fragrant.

2. Add curry powder and cumin, cooking for 1 minute.

3. Stir in lentils, sweet potatoes, vegetable broth, and coconut milk. Bring to a boil, then reduce heat and simmer for 25-30 minutes until lentils and sweet potatoes are tender.

4. Season with salt and pepper before serving.

Nutrition Information (per serving):

- Calories: 320
- Protein: 11g
- Carbohydrates: 48g
- Fat: 12g
- Fiber: 10g
- Sugar: 8g
- Portion Size: 1 cup

Baked Eggplant Parmesan

Ingredients:

- 1 large eggplant, sliced into rounds
- 2 cups marinara sauce
- 1 cup shredded mozzarella cheese
- 1/2 cup grated Parmesan cheese
- 1 cup whole wheat breadcrumbs
- 2 eggs, beaten
- 1/2 cup flour

- 2 tbsp olive oil
- Salt and pepper to taste

Instructions:

1. Preheat oven to 375°F (190°C).
2. Season eggplant slices with salt and let sit for 10 minutes. Pat dry.
3. Dredge each slice in flour, dip in beaten eggs, and coat with breadcrumbs.
4. Heat olive oil in a pan over medium heat. Fry eggplant slices until golden brown.
5. In a baking dish, layer fried eggplant, marinara sauce, mozzarella, and Parmesan cheese. Repeat layers.
6. Bake for 25-30 minutes until cheese is bubbly and golden brown.

Nutrition Information (per serving):

- Calories: 350
- Protein: 14g
- Carbohydrates: 38g
- Fat: 16g
- Fiber: 8g
- Sugar: 10g
- Portion Size: 1 cup

Chapter 5: Snacks and Appetizers

Snacks and appetizers play a crucial role in a balanced diet, providing opportunities to incorporate nutrients while satisfying cravings between meals. These recipes are designed to be wholesome, delicious, and easy to prepare, making them perfect for any occasion from a casual gathering to a quick afternoon pick-me-up.

Hummus and Veggie Platter

Ingredients:

- 1 cup hummus
- Assorted fresh vegetables (carrots, cucumbers, bell peppers, cherry tomatoes)

Instructions:

1. Arrange the hummus in the center of a platter.
2. Surround the hummus with sliced vegetables.
3. Serve immediately.

Nutrition Information (per serving):

- Calories: 150
- Protein: 6g

- Carbohydrates: 18g

- Fat: 7g

- Fiber: 6g

- Sugar: 4g

- Portion size: 1/2 cup hummus with vegetables

Spicy Roasted Chickpeas

Ingredients:

- 1 can (15 oz) chickpeas, drained and rinsed

- 1 tbsp olive oil

- 1 tsp smoked paprika

- 1/2 tsp cayenne pepper

- Salt to taste

Instructions:

1. Preheat oven to 400°F (200°C).

2. Pat dry chickpeas with paper towels to remove excess moisture.

3. Toss chickpeas with olive oil, smoked paprika, cayenne pepper, and salt.

4. Spread chickpeas in a single layer on a baking sheet.

5. Roast for 25-30 minutes, stirring halfway through, until crispy.

6. Let cool before serving.

Nutrition Information (per serving):

- Calories: 180
- Protein: 7g
- Carbohydrates: 25g
- Fat: 6g
- Fiber: 7g
- Sugar: 4g
- Portion size: 1/2 cup

Avocado and Black Bean Salsa

Ingredients:

- 1 ripe avocado, diced
- 1 cup black beans, drained and rinsed
- 1/2 cup diced tomatoes
- 1/4 cup diced red onion
- 1/4 cup chopped cilantro
- Juice of 1 lime
- Salt and pepper to taste

Instructions:

1. In a bowl, combine avocado, black beans, tomatoes, red onion, and cilantro.
2. Drizzle lime juice over the mixture and gently toss.
3. Season with salt and pepper.
4. Serve chilled with whole grain tortilla chips or as a topping for salads.

Nutrition Information (per serving):

- Calories: 160
- Protein: 6g
- Carbohydrates: 22g
- Fat: 7g
- Fiber: 8g
- Sugar: 1g
- Portion size: 1/2 cup

Greek Yogurt with Berries and Honey

Ingredients:

- 1 cup Greek yogurt
- 1/2 cup mixed berries (such as blueberries, strawberries, raspberries)
- 1 tbsp honey

Instructions:

1. Spoon Greek yogurt into a serving bowl.
2. Top with mixed berries.
3. Drizzle honey over the berries.
4. Serve immediately.

Nutrition Information (per serving):

- Calories: 180
- Protein: 18g
- Carbohydrates: 25g
- Fat: 2g
- Fiber: 3g
- Sugar: 19g
- Portion size: 1 cup

Mini Caprese Skewers

Ingredients:

- Cherry tomatoes
- Fresh mozzarella balls
- Fresh basil leaves
- Balsamic glaze (optional)
- Salt and pepper to taste

Instructions:

1. Thread a cherry tomato, a small mozzarella ball, and a basil leaf onto each skewer.
2. Arrange on a serving platter.
3. Drizzle with balsamic glaze if desired.
4. Season with salt and pepper.
5. Serve immediately.

Nutrition Information (per serving, 2 skewers):

- Calories: 120
- Protein: 7g
- Carbohydrates: 3g
- Fat: 9g
- Fiber: 1g
- Sugar: 1g
- Portion size: 2 skewers

Edamame with Sea Salt

Ingredients:

- 2 cups edamame (frozen, thawed)
- Sea salt, to taste

Instructions:

1. Bring a pot of water to a boil.

2. Add edamame and cook for 3-4 minutes until tender.

3. Drain and rinse with cold water.

4. Sprinkle with sea salt.

5. Serve immediately.

Nutrition Information (per serving):

- Calories: 150

- Protein: 13g

- Carbohydrates: 11g

- Fat: 6g

- Fiber: 8g

- Sugar: 3g

- Portion size: 1 cup

Almond Butter Stuffed Dates

Ingredients:

- Medjool dates, pitted

- Almond butter

Instructions:

1. Carefully slit dates lengthwise and remove pits.

2. Fill each date with almond butter.

3. Serve immediately or chill before serving.

Nutrition Information (per serving, 2 dates):

- Calories: 160

- Protein: 4g

- Carbohydrates: 28g

- Fat: 6g

- Fiber: 4g

- Sugar: 24g

- Portion size: 2 dates

Baked Zucchini Fries

Ingredients:

- 2 zucchinis, cut into sticks

- 1/2 cup breadcrumbs (whole wheat if possible)

- 1/4 cup grated Parmesan cheese

- 1 tsp garlic powder

- Salt and pepper to taste

- Olive oil spray

Instructions:

1. Preheat oven to 425°F (220°C). Line a baking sheet with parchment paper.
2. In a bowl, combine breadcrumbs, Parmesan cheese, garlic powder, salt, and pepper.
3. Dip zucchini sticks into the breadcrumb mixture, coating evenly.
4. Place on the baking sheet and lightly spray with olive oil.
5. Bake for 20-25 minutes, turning halfway through, until golden brown and crispy.
6. Serve hot with marinara sauce or a yogurt-based dip.

Nutrition Information (per serving):

- Calories: 140
- Protein: 6g
- Carbohydrates: 18g
- Fat: 6g
- Fiber: 3g
- Sugar: 4g
- Portion size: 1 cup

Guacamole with Carrot and Celery Sticks

Ingredients:

- 2 ripe avocados
- 1 tomato, diced
- 1/4 cup diced red onion
- 1/4 cup chopped cilantro
- Juice of 1 lime
- Salt and pepper to taste
- Carrot and celery sticks, for serving

Instructions:

1. Scoop avocado flesh into a bowl and mash with a fork.
2. Add diced tomato, red onion, cilantro, lime juice, salt, and pepper.
3. Mix until well combined.
4. Serve guacamole with carrot and celery sticks.

Nutrition Information (per serving, 1/4 cup guacamole with sticks):

- Calories: 160
- Protein: 3g
- Carbohydrates: 12g
- Fat: 13g
- Fiber: 7g
- Sugar: 2g

*   Portion size: 1/4 cup guacamole with sticks

Fresh Fruit and Nut Mix

Ingredients:

*   Assorted fresh fruits (such as grapes, apple slices, berries)
*   Mixed nuts (almonds, walnuts, cashews)

Instructions:

1. Combine fresh fruits and mixed nuts in a bowl.
2. Toss gently to mix.
3. Serve immediately.

Nutrition Information (per serving):

*   Calories: 180
*   Protein: 5g
*   Carbohydrates: 22g
*   Fat: 10g
*   Fiber: 5g
*   Sugar: 14g
*   Portion size: 1 cup

Cottage Cheese and Pineapple Bites

Ingredients:

- Cottage cheese
- Fresh pineapple, cubed

Instructions:

1. Scoop cottage cheese into bite-sized portions.
2. Top each portion with a cube of fresh pineapple.
3. Serve chilled or at room temperature.

Nutrition Information (per serving, 1/2):

- Calories: 120
- Protein: 12g
- Carbohydrates: 15g
- Fat: 2g
- Fiber: 1g
- Sugar: 12g
- Portion size: 1/2 cup cottage cheese with pineapple

Spinach and Artichoke Dip with Whole Grain Crackers

Ingredients:

- 1 cup frozen spinach, thawed and drained

- 1 can (14 oz) artichoke hearts, drained and chopped
- 1 cup plain Greek yogurt
- 1/2 cup grated Parmesan cheese
- 1/2 cup shredded mozzarella cheese
- 1/2 tsp garlic powder
- Salt and pepper to taste
- Whole grain crackers, for serving

Instructions:

1. Preheat oven to 375°F (190°C).
2. In a bowl, combine thawed spinach, chopped artichoke hearts, Greek yogurt, Parmesan cheese, mozzarella cheese, garlic powder, salt, and pepper.
3. Transfer mixture to a baking dish.
4. Bake for 20-25 minutes, until bubbly and golden brown on top.
5. Serve warm with whole grain crackers.

Nutrition Information (per serving, 1/4 cup dip with crackers):

- Calories: 160
- Protein: 10g
- Carbohydrates: 12g
- Fat: 8g
- Fiber: 3g

- Sugar: 2g

- Portion size: 1/4 cup dip with crackers

Cucumber and Hummus Roll-Ups

Ingredients:

- 1 large cucumber

- Hummus

- Cherry tomatoes, halved (optional)

- Fresh herbs (such as parsley or cilantro), for garnish

Instructions:

1. Use a vegetable peeler to slice the cucumber lengthwise into thin strips.

2. Spread a thin layer of hummus on each cucumber strip.

3. Place a cherry tomato half (if using) at one end of each strip.

4. Roll up tightly.

5. Secure with a toothpick if needed.

6. Garnish with fresh herbs.

7. Serve chilled.

Nutrition Information (per serving, 4 roll-ups):

- Calories: 100

- Protein: 4g

- Carbohydrates: 14g

- Fat: 4g

- Fiber: 4g

- Sugar: 4g

- Portion size: 4 roll-ups

Tomato Basil Bruschetta

Ingredients:

- 4-5 ripe tomatoes, diced

- 1/4 cup fresh basil leaves, chopped

- 2 cloves garlic, minced

- 2 tbsp extra virgin olive oil

- 1 tbsp balsamic vinegar

- Salt and pepper to taste

- Slices of whole grain baguette, toasted

Instructions:

1. In a bowl, combine diced tomatoes, chopped basil, minced garlic, olive oil, balsamic vinegar, salt, and pepper.

2. Mix well and let it sit for 10-15 minutes to allow flavors to meld.

3. Spoon tomato mixture onto toasted whole grain baguette slices.

4. Serve immediately.

Nutrition Information (per serving, 2 slices of bruschetta):

- Calories: 160
- Protein: 4g
- Carbohydrates: 20g
- Fat: 7g
- Fiber: 3g
- Sugar: 4g
- Portion size: 2 slices of bruschetta

Mixed Nuts and Seeds Trail Mix

Ingredients:

- 1 cup mixed nuts (almonds, walnuts, cashews)
- 1/2 cup mixed seeds (pumpkin seeds, sunflower seeds)
- 1/4 cup dried fruits (cranberries, raisins, apricots)
- 1/4 tsp sea salt (optional)

Instructions:

1. In a bowl, combine mixed nuts, mixed seeds, and dried fruits.
2. Add sea salt if desired.
3. Toss well to mix evenly.

4. Portion into individual servings or store in an airtight container for later use.

Nutrition Information (per serving, 1/4 cup):

- Calories: 200
- Protein: 6g
- Carbohydrates: 15g
- Fat: 14g
- Fiber: 4g
- Sugar: 8g
- Portion size: 1/4 cup

Chapter 6: Desserts

These recipes are crafted with wholesome ingredients to support your health goals without compromising on flavor. Each dessert is not only delicious but also provides essential nutritional information to help you make informed choices. Enjoy these treats guilt-free as part of your balanced diet.

Berry Chia Seed Pudding

Ingredients:

- 1/4 cup chia seeds
- 1 cup unsweetened almond milk
- 1/2 teaspoon vanilla extract
- 1 tablespoon maple syrup
- 1/2 cup mixed berries

Instructions:

1. In a bowl, mix chia seeds, almond milk, vanilla extract, and maple syrup.
2. Stir well and refrigerate for at least 2 hours or overnight.
3. Top with mixed berries before serving.

Nutrition Information:

- Calories: 180
- Protein: 5g
- Carbohydrates: 20g
- Fat: 9g
- Fiber: 10g
- Sugar: 7g
- Portion size: 1 serving

Baked Apple with Cinnamon and Walnuts

Ingredients:

- 1 apple, cored
- 1 tablespoon chopped walnuts
- 1/2 teaspoon cinnamon
- 1 teaspoon honey

Instructions:

1. Preheat oven to 375°F (190°C).
2. Place cored apple on a baking sheet.
3. Fill the center with chopped walnuts and sprinkle with cinnamon.

4. Drizzle honey over the top and bake for 20-25 minutes until tender.

Nutrition Information:

- Calories: 150
- Protein: 2g
- Carbohydrates: 25g
- Fat: 6g
- Fiber: 5g
- Sugar: 18g
- Portion size: 1 apple

Dark Chocolate Avocado Mousse

Ingredients:

- 1 ripe avocado
- 2 tablespoons cocoa powder
- 2 tablespoons maple syrup
- 1/2 teaspoon vanilla extract
- Dark chocolate shavings for garnish (optional)

Instructions:

1. In a food processor, blend avocado until smooth.

2. Add cocoa powder, maple syrup, and vanilla extract. Blend until creamy.

3. Chill in the refrigerator for 30 minutes before serving.

4. Garnish with dark chocolate shavings if desired.

Nutrition Information:

- Calories: 200
- Protein: 3g
- Carbohydrates: 18g
- Fat: 14g
- Fiber: 7g
- Sugar: 8g
- Portion size: 1 serving

Coconut Mango Chia Pudding

Ingredients:

- 1/4 cup chia seeds
- 1 cup coconut milk
- 1 tablespoon maple syrup
- 1/2 cup diced mango

Instructions:

1. In a bowl, combine chia seeds, coconut milk, and maple syrup.
2. Stir well and refrigerate for at least 4 hours or overnight.
3. Top with diced mango before serving.

Nutrition Information:

- Calories: 220
- Protein: 5g
- Carbohydrates: 25g
- Fat: 12g
- Fiber: 10g
- Sugar: 10g
- Portion size: 1 serving

Grilled Peaches with Honey and Yogurt

Ingredients:

- 2 peaches, halved and pitted
- 1 tablespoon honey
- Greek yogurt for serving
- Fresh mint leaves for garnish

Instructions:

1. Preheat grill or grill pan over medium heat.

2. Grill peach halves for 2-3 minutes on each side until grill marks appear.

3. Drizzle with honey and serve with a dollop of Greek yogurt.

4. Garnish with fresh mint leaves.

Nutrition Information:

- Calories: 120

- Protein: 4g

- Carbohydrates: 25g

- Fat: 1g

- Fiber: 3g

- Sugar: 20g

- Portion size: 1 peach

Vegan Chocolate Chip Cookies

Ingredients:

- 1 cup almond flour

- 1/4 cup coconut oil, melted

- 1/4 cup maple syrup

- 1/2 teaspoon vanilla extract

- 1/4 cup dairy-free chocolate chips

Instructions:

1. Preheat oven to 350°F (175°C) and line a baking sheet with parchment paper.
2. In a bowl, mix almond flour, melted coconut oil, maple syrup, and vanilla extract until dough forms.
3. Fold in chocolate chips.
4. Form dough into tablespoon-sized balls and place on the baking sheet.
5. Flatten each ball with a fork.
6. Bake for 10-12 minutes until edges are golden brown.
7. Allow to cool before serving.

Nutrition Information:

- Calories: 150
- Protein: 3g
- Carbohydrates: 12g
- Fat: 10g
- Fiber: 2g
- Sugar: 8g
- Portion size: 2 cookies

Banana Nice Cream

Ingredients:

- 2 ripe bananas, sliced and frozen
- 1 tablespoon almond milk (if needed for blending)

Instructions:

1. Place frozen banana slices in a blender or food processor.
2. Blend until smooth and creamy, adding almond milk if necessary.
3. Serve immediately as soft-serve consistency, or freeze for 30 minutes for a firmer texture.

Nutrition Information:

- Calories: 120
- Protein: 1g
- Carbohydrates: 31g
- Fat: 0.5g
- Fiber: 3g
- Sugar: 18g
- Portion size: 1 serving

Almond Butter Brownies

Ingredients:

- 1/2 cup almond butter
- 1/4 cup cocoa powder
- 1/4 cup maple syrup
- 1/2 teaspoon baking powder
- 1/4 teaspoon salt
- 1/4 cup dairy-free chocolate chips (optional)

Instructions:

1. Preheat oven to 350°F (175°C) and grease a baking dish.
2. In a bowl, mix almond butter, cocoa powder, maple syrup, baking powder, and salt until smooth.
3. Fold in chocolate chips, if using.
4. Spread batter evenly into the prepared baking dish.
5. Bake for 20-25 minutes until edges are set.
6. Allow to cool before cutting into squares.

Nutrition Information:

- Calories: 180
- Protein: 5g
- Carbohydrates: 20g
- Fat: 10g
- Fiber: 3g

- Sugar: 12g

- Portion size: 1 brownie

Chilled Coconut Rice Pudding

Ingredients:

- 1/2 cup jasmine rice

- 1 can (14 oz) coconut milk

- 2 tablespoons maple syrup

- 1/2 teaspoon vanilla extract

- Fresh berries for topping

Instructions:

1. Cook jasmine rice according to package instructions and let it cool.

2. In a saucepan, combine coconut milk, maple syrup, and vanilla extract. Heat until warm.

3. Stir in cooked rice and simmer for 15-20 minutes until creamy.

4. Remove from heat and let cool.

5. Serve chilled topped with fresh berries.

Nutrition Information:

- Calories: 250

- Protein: 3g

- Carbohydrates: 30g

- Fat: 14g

- Fiber: 1g

- Sugar: 8g

- Portion size: 1 serving

Fresh Berry Salad with Mint

Ingredients:

- 1 cup mixed fresh berries (strawberries, blueberries, raspberries)
- 1 tablespoon fresh mint leaves, chopped
- 1 teaspoon honey or maple syrup (optional)

Instructions:

1. Wash and prepare the berries as needed.
2. In a bowl, gently toss together mixed berries and chopped mint leaves.
3. Drizzle with honey or maple syrup if desired.
4. Serve immediately.

Nutrition Information:

- Calories: 50

- Protein: 1g

- Carbohydrates: 12g

- Fat: 0.5g

- Fiber: 4g

- Sugar: 8g

- Portion size: 1 serving

Apple and Oat Crumble

Ingredients:

- 2 apples, peeled and sliced

- 1 tablespoon lemon juice

- 1/2 cup rolled oats

- 1/4 cup almond flour

- 2 tablespoons coconut oil, melted

- 2 tablespoons maple syrup

- 1/2 teaspoon cinnamon

Instructions:

1. Preheat oven to 350°F (175°C) and grease a baking dish.

2. Toss apple slices with lemon juice and spread evenly in the baking dish.

3. In a bowl, mix rolled oats, almond flour, melted coconut oil, maple syrup, and cinnamon until crumbly.

4. Spread oat mixture over the apples.

5. Bake for 30-35 minutes until topping is golden brown and apples are tender.

6. Allow to cool slightly before serving.

Nutrition Information:

- Calories: 200

- Protein: 3g

- Carbohydrates: 30g

- Fat: 8g

- Fiber: 5g

- Sugar: 16g

- Portion size: 1 serving

Pumpkin Spice Energy Balls

Ingredients:

- 1 cup rolled oats

- 1/2 cup pumpkin puree

- 1/4 cup almond butter

- 2 tablespoons maple syrup

- 1 teaspoon pumpkin pie spice

- 1/4 cup chopped nuts (optional)

Instructions:

1. In a bowl, combine rolled oats, pumpkin puree, almond butter, maple syrup, and pumpkin pie spice until well mixed.
2. Fold in chopped nuts if desired.
3. Roll mixture into tablespoon-sized balls and place on a baking sheet lined with parchment paper.
4. Chill in the refrigerator for at least 30 minutes before serving.

Nutrition Information:

- Calories: 120
- Protein: 4g
- Carbohydrates: 15g
- Fat: 6g
- Fiber: 3g
- Sugar: 5g
- Portion size: 2 balls

Raw Cashew Cheesecake Bites

Ingredients:

- 1 cup raw cashews, soaked in water for 4 hours or overnight
- 1/4 cup coconut oil, melted
- 1/4 cup maple syrup

- 1/4 cup lemon juice
- 1 teaspoon vanilla extract
- Fresh berries for garnish

Instructions:

1. Drain soaked cashews and place them in a food processor or blender.
2. Add melted coconut oil, maple syrup, lemon juice, and vanilla extract.
3. Blend until smooth and creamy, scraping down the sides as needed.
4. Line a mini muffin tin with paper liners.
5. Spoon cashew mixture into each liner, filling almost to the top.
6. Chill in the freezer for at least 2 hours until set.
7. Remove from freezer, garnish with fresh berries, and serve chilled.

Nutrition Information:

- Calories: 150
- Protein: 3g
- Carbohydrates: 12g
- Fat: 10g
- Fiber: 1g

- Sugar: 8g
- Portion size: 2 bites

Lemon Blueberry Bars

Ingredients:

- 1 cup almond flour
- 1/4 cup coconut flour
- 1/4 cup coconut oil, melted
- 1/4 cup maple syrup
- Zest and juice of 1 lemon
- 1 cup fresh or frozen blueberries

Instructions:

1. Preheat oven to 350°F (175°C) and line a baking dish with parchment paper.
2. In a bowl, mix almond flour, coconut flour, melted coconut oil, maple syrup, lemon zest, and lemon juice until dough forms.
3. Press half of the dough evenly into the bottom of the baking dish.
4. Scatter blueberries over the dough.
5. Crumble the remaining dough over the blueberries.
6. Bake for 25-30 minutes until edges are golden brown.

7. Allow to cool completely before cutting into bars.

Nutrition Information:

- Calories: 180
- Protein: 3g
- Carbohydrates: 20g
- Fat: 10g
- Fiber: 3g
- Sugar: 10g
- Portion size: 1 bar

Chocolate Dipped Strawberries

Ingredients:

- 1 cup dark chocolate chips
- 1 tablespoon coconut oil
- 12 fresh strawberries, washed and dried

Instructions:

1. In a microwave-safe bowl, melt dark chocolate chips and coconut oil in 30-second intervals, stirring in between, until smooth.
2. Dip each strawberry into the melted chocolate, letting excess drip off.

3. Place dipped strawberries on a parchment-lined baking sheet.

4. Refrigerate for 15-20 minutes until chocolate sets.

Nutrition Information:

- Calories: 150
- Protein: 2g
- Carbohydrates: 20g
- Fat: 9g
- Fiber: 4g
- Sugar: 14g
- Portion size: 2 strawberries

Chapter 7: Smoothies

They can be enjoyed as a quick breakfast, a satisfying snack, or even a light meal replacement. Each smoothie in this chapter is carefully crafted to balance flavors and nutritional benefits, providing a delicious way to support your health goals. From antioxidant-rich berries to creamy avocado, each recipe offers a unique blend of flavors and textures that are sure to delight your taste buds while supporting your journey towards better health.

Green Detox Smoothie

Ingredients:

- 1 cup spinach
- 1/2 cucumber, peeled and chopped
- 1/2 green apple, chopped
- 1/2 lemon, juiced
- 1/2 cup coconut water
- Ice cubes, as desired

Instructions:

1. Place all ingredients in a blender.
2. Blend until smooth.
3. Serve immediately.

Nutrition Information:

- Calories: 90
- Protein: 3g
- Carbohydrates: 21g
- Fat: 1g
- Fiber: 5g
- Sugar: 12g
- Portion Size: 1 serving

Strawberry Banana Protein Smoothie

Ingredients:

- 1 cup strawberries, hulled
- 1 ripe banana
- 1/2 cup Greek yogurt
- 1 scoop vanilla protein powder
- 1/2 cup almond milk
- Ice cubes, as desired

Instructions:

1. Combine all ingredients in a blender.
2. Blend until smooth and creamy.
3. Enjoy immediately.

Nutrition Information:

- Calories: 280
- Protein: 25g
- Carbohydrates: 40g
- Fat: 3g
- Fiber: 7g
- Sugar: 23g
- Portion Size: 1 serving

Tropical Mango and Pineapple Smoothie

Ingredients:

- 1 cup frozen mango chunks
- 1 cup fresh pineapple chunks
- 1/2 cup coconut milk
- 1/2 cup orange juice
- 1 tbsp honey or agave syrup (optional)
- Ice cubes, as desired

Instructions:

1. Place mango, pineapple, coconut milk, orange juice, and honey (if using) in a blender.
2. Blend until smooth and creamy.
3. Serve immediately.

Nutrition Information:

- Calories: 220
- Protein: 2g
- Carbohydrates: 52g
- Fat: 3g
- Fiber: 4g
- Sugar: 42g
- Portion Size: 1 serving

Spinach and Kiwi Smoothie

Ingredients:

- 1 cup fresh spinach
- 2 kiwis, peeled and chopped
- 1/2 cup plain Greek yogurt
- 1/2 cup almond milk
- 1 tbsp honey or maple syrup (optional)
- Ice cubes, as desired

Instructions:

1. Combine spinach, kiwis, Greek yogurt, almond milk, and honey (if using) in a blender.
2. Blend until smooth.
3. Serve immediately.

Nutrition Information:

- Calories: 160
- Protein: 7g
- Carbohydrates: 30g
- Fat: 3g
- Fiber: 5g
- Sugar: 20g
- Portion Size: 1 serving

Blueberry Almond Butter Smoothie

Ingredients:

- 1 cup frozen blueberries
- 1 tbsp almond butter
- 1/2 cup Greek yogurt
- 1/2 cup almond milk
- 1 tbsp honey or agave syrup (optional)
- Ice cubes, as desired

Instructions:

1. Place blueberries, almond butter, Greek yogurt, almond milk, and honey (if using) in a blender.
2. Blend until smooth.
3. Enjoy immediately.

Nutrition Information:

- Calories: 250
- Protein: 12g
- Carbohydrates: 35g
- Fat: 8g
- Fiber: 6g
- Sugar: 24g
- Portion Size: 1 serving

Avocado and Cucumber Smoothie

Ingredients:

- 1/2 ripe avocado
- 1/2 cucumber, peeled and chopped
- 1 cup spinach
- 1/2 cup coconut water
- Juice of 1 lime
- Ice cubes, as desired

Instructions:

1. Combine avocado, cucumber, spinach, coconut water, and lime juice in a blender.
2. Blend until smooth and creamy.
3. Serve chilled.

Nutrition Information:

- Calories: 180
- Protein: 4g
- Carbohydrates: 20g
- Fat: 11g
- Fiber: 8g
- Sugar: 7g
- Portion Size: 1 serving

Peanut Butter and Banana Smoothie

Ingredients:

- 1 ripe banana
- 2 tbsp peanut butter
- 1/2 cup Greek yogurt
- 1/2 cup almond milk
- 1 tbsp honey or maple syrup (optional)
- Ice cubes, as desired

Instructions:

1. Combine banana, peanut butter, Greek yogurt, almond milk, and honey (if using) in a blender.
2. Blend until smooth and creamy.
3. Serve immediately.

Nutrition Information:

- Calories: 300
- Protein: 15g
- Carbohydrates: 35g
- Fat: 12g
- Fiber: 5g
- Sugar: 20g
- Portion Size: 1 serving

Raspberry and Chia Seed Smoothie

Ingredients:

- 1 cup raspberries (fresh or frozen)
- 1 tbsp chia seeds
- 1/2 cup plain Greek yogurt
- 1/2 cup almond milk
- 1 tbsp honey or agave syrup (optional)
- Ice cubes, as desired

Instructions:

1. Place raspberries, chia seeds, Greek yogurt, almond milk, and honey (if using) in a blender.
2. Blend until smooth.
3. Enjoy immediately.

Nutrition Information:

- Calories: 200
- Protein: 9g
- Carbohydrates: 30g
- Fat: 6g
- Fiber: 10g
- Sugar: 15g
- Portion Size: 1 serving

Carrot and Ginger Smoothie

Ingredients:

- 1 large carrot, peeled and chopped
- 1-inch piece of fresh ginger, peeled and grated
- 1/2 cup plain Greek yogurt
- 1/2 cup almond milk
- 1 tbsp honey or maple syrup (optional)
- Ice cubes, as desired

Instructions:

1. Combine carrot, ginger, Greek yogurt, almond milk, and honey (if using) in a blender.
2. Blend until smooth.
3. Serve chilled.

Nutrition Information:

- Calories: 180
- Protein: 8g
- Carbohydrates: 30g
- Fat: 3g
- Fiber: 5g
- Sugar: 20g
- Portion Size: 1 serving

Chocolate Cherry Smoothie

Ingredients:

- 1 cup frozen cherries
- 1 tbsp cocoa powder
- 1/2 cup Greek yogurt
- 1/2 cup almond milk
- 1 tbsp honey or agave syrup (optional)
- Ice cubes, as desired

Instructions:

1. Combine cherries, cocoa powder, Greek yogurt, almond milk, and honey (if using) in a blender.
2. Blend until smooth and creamy.
3. Serve immediately.

Nutrition Information:

- Calories: 230
- Protein: 10g
- Carbohydrates: 40g
- Fat: 5g
- Fiber: 6g
- Sugar: 30g
- Portion Size: 1 serving

Pineapple and Kale Smoothie

Ingredients:

- 1 cup fresh kale leaves, stems removed
- 1 cup frozen pineapple chunks
- 1/2 cup coconut water
- Juice of 1/2 lime
- 1 tbsp honey or agave syrup (optional)
- Ice cubes, as desired

Instructions:

1. Combine kale, pineapple, coconut water, lime juice, and honey (if using) in a blender.
2. Blend until smooth and creamy.
3. Enjoy immediately.

Nutrition Information:

- Calories: 150
- Protein: 3g
- Carbohydrates: 35g
- Fat: 1g
- Fiber: 5g
- Sugar: 20g
- Portion Size: 1 serving

Berry Beet Smoothie

Ingredients:

- 1/2 cup cooked beets, chopped
- 1/2 cup mixed berries (such as strawberries, blueberries, raspberries)
- 1/2 cup plain Greek yogurt
- 1/2 cup almond milk
- 1 tbsp honey or maple syrup (optional)
- Ice cubes, as desired

Instructions:

1. Combine beets, mixed berries, Greek yogurt, almond milk, and honey (if using) in a blender.
2. Blend until smooth and vibrant.

3. Serve chilled.

Nutrition Information:

- Calories: 200

- Protein: 10g

- Carbohydrates: 35g

- Fat: 3g

- Fiber: 6g

- Sugar: 25g

- Portion Size: 1 serving

Apple Cinnamon Smoothie

Ingredients:

- 1 apple, cored and chopped

- 1/2 tsp ground cinnamon

- 1/2 cup plain Greek yogurt

- 1/2 cup almond milk

- 1 tbsp honey or maple syrup (optional)

- Ice cubes, as desired

Instructions:

1. Combine apple, cinnamon, Greek yogurt, almond milk, and honey (if using) in a blender.

2. Blend until smooth and creamy.

3. Serve immediately.

Nutrition Information:

- Calories: 180

- Protein: 8g

- Carbohydrates: 35g

- Fat: 3g

- Fiber: 5g

- Sugar: 25g

- Portion Size: 1 serving

Matcha Green Tea Smoothie

Ingredients:

- 1 tsp matcha green tea powder

- 1 banana

- 1/2 cup spinach

- 1/2 cup plain Greek yogurt

- 1/2 cup almond milk

- Ice cubes, as desired

Instructions:

1. Blend matcha green tea powder, banana, spinach, Greek yogurt, and almond milk until smooth.
2. Serve immediately.

Nutrition Information:

- Calories: 200
- Protein: 10g
- Carbohydrates: 35g
- Fat: 3g
- Fiber: 5g
- Sugar: 20g
- Portion Size: 1 serving

Orange and Carrot Sunshine Smoothie

Ingredients:

- 1 orange, peeled and segmented
- 1 large carrot, peeled and chopped
- 1/2 cup plain Greek yogurt
- 1/2 cup almond milk
- 1 tbsp honey or agave syrup (optional)
- Ice cubes, as desired

Instructions:

1. Combine orange segments, chopped carrot, Greek yogurt, almond milk, and honey (if using) in a blender.
2. Blend until smooth and creamy.
3. Serve chilled.

Nutrition Information:

- Calories: 180
- Protein: 8g
- Carbohydrates: 35g
- Fat: 3g
- Fiber: 5g
- Sugar: 25g
- Portion Size: 1 serving

CONCLUSION

Congratulations on completing "Prediabetes Vegetarian Recipes for Weight Loss"! This cookbook has been crafted with your health and well-being in mind, offering a diverse array of delicious vegetarian recipes designed specifically to help manage prediabetes and support weight loss goals.

Throughout this journey, you've explored the power of nutrition in managing prediabetes, discovering how a plant-based diet can make a significant difference in stabilizing blood sugar levels and promoting overall health. From hearty breakfasts to satisfying dinners, refreshing smoothies to tempting desserts, each recipe has been thoughtfully curated to ensure balanced nutrition without sacrificing flavor.

As you move forward, remember that this cookbook is more than just a collection of recipes—it's a guide to adopting sustainable dietary habits. By incorporating these nutrient-dense meals into your daily routine, you're not only taking proactive steps toward managing prediabetes but also cultivating a healthier lifestyle for the long term.

Continue to experiment with flavors, explore new ingredients, and enjoy the process of nourishing your body with wholesome foods. Embrace mindful eating practices, stay active, and seek support from healthcare professionals as needed to achieve your health goals.

Thank you for embarking on this journey with us. Here's to your health, vitality, and the joy of flavorful, nutritious meals!